THE EASY DIABETIC COOKBOOK FOR BEGINNERS

How to Lose Weight and Stay Healthy with Delicious Recipes from Breakfast to Dinner

Sophie Kruis

© Copyright 2021 By Sophie Kruis - All rights reserved.

The content contained within this book may not be reproduced, duplicated or transmitted without direct written permission from the author or the publisher.

Under no circumstances will any blame or legal responsibility be held against the publisher, or author, for any damages, reparation, or monetary loss due to the information contained within this book. Either directly or indirectly.

Legal Notice:

This book is copyright protected. This book is only for personal use. You cannot amend, distribute, sell, use, quote or paraphrase any part, or the content within this book, without the consent of the author or publisher.

Disclaimer Notice:

Please note the information contained within this document is for educational and entertainment purposes only. All effort has been executed to present accurate, up to date, and reliable, complete information. No warranties of any kind are declared or implied. Readers acknowledge that the author is not engaging in the rendering of legal, financial, medical or professional advice. The content within this book has been derived from various sources. Please consult a licensed professional before attempting any techniques outlined in this book.

By reading this document, the reader agrees that under no circumstances is the author responsible for any losses, direct or indirect, which are incurred as a result of the use of information contained within this document, including, but not limited to, errors, omissions, or inaccuracies.

Table Of Contents

INTRODUCTION 7

BREAKFAST RECIPES 10
1. CREAMED SPINACH 10
2. STUFFED MUSHROOMS 12
3. BERRY-OAT BREAKFAST BARS 14
4. WHOLE-GRAIN BREAKFAST COOKIES 16

APPETIZER RECIPES 19
5. BROCCOLI SALAD 19
6. CHICKEN SALAD IN CUCUMBER CUPS 21
7. SUNFLOWER SEEDS AND ARUGULA GARDEN SALAD 22
8. SUPREME CAESAR SALAD 23
9. TABBOULEH- ARABIAN SALAD 25
10. AROMATIC TOASTED PUMPKIN SEEDS 27
11. BACON-WRAPPED SHRIMPS 29

FIRST COURSE RECIPES 31
12. ITALIAN BEEF 31
13. LAMB WITH BROCCOLI & CARROTS 33
14. ROSEMARY LAMB 35
15. MEDITERRANEAN LAMB MEATBALLS 37

SECOND COURSE RECIPES 39
16. CRAB FRITTATA 39
17. CRUNCHY LEMON SHRIMP 41
18. GRILLED TUNA STEAKS 43
19. RED CLAM SAUCE & PASTA 45
20. SALMON MILANO 47
21. SHRIMP & ARTICHOKE SKILLET 48
22. TUNA CARBONARA 49
23. MEDITERRANEAN FISH FILLETS 51

SIDE DISH RECIPES 54
24. CHIA CRACKERS 54
25. ORANGE- SPICED PUMPKIN HUMMUS 56
26. CINNAMON MAPLE SWEET POTATO BITES 57
27. CHEESY KALE CHIPS 59

28.	LEMON ROASTED BELL PEPPER	61
29.	SUBTLE ROASTED MUSHROOMS	62
30.	FANCY SPELT BREAD	64
31.	CRISPY CRUNCHY HUMMUS	66

SOUPS & STEWS 68

32.	CREAMY LENTIL AND POTATO STEW	68
33.	ROASTED GARLIC AND CAULIFLOWER SOUP	70
34.	BEEFLESS "BEEF" STEW	72
35.	CREAMY MUSHROOM SOUP	74
36.	CHILLED BERRY AND MINT SOUP	76
37.	VEGETABLE SOUP	78

DESSERTS 81

38.	WALNUT-FRUIT CAKE	81
39.	GINGER CAKE	83
40.	KETOGENIC ORANGE CAKE	85
41.	LEMON CAKE	88
42.	CINNAMON CAKE	90
43.	BANANA NUT MUFFINS	93
44.	MANGO NUT CHEESECAKE	95

JUICE AND SMOOTHIE RECIPES 97

45.	STRAWBERRY – ORANGE SMOOTHIES (SOS)	97
46.	TAMARIND – PEAR SMOOTHIE (TPS)	99
47.	CURRANT ELDERBERRY SMOOTHIE (CES)	101
48.	SWEET DREAM STRAWBERRY SMOOTHIE	103
49.	ALKALINE GREEN GINGER AND BANANA CLEANSING SMOOTHIE	105
50.	ORANGE MIXED DETOX SMOOTHIE	106
51.	CUCUMBER TOXIN FLUSH SMOOTHIE	107

CONCLUSION 109

Introduction

Diabetes is a condition in which the body is no longer able to self-regulate blood glucose. When you eat a food that contains carbohydrates, whether it's honey, an apple, or brown rice, your body breaks it down into sugar (also called glucose) during digestion. This glucose passes through the walls of the intestines into the bloodstream, which causes blood sugar (the amount of glucose circulating in the blood) to rise.

In response, the pancreas secretes a hormone called insulin. Insulin's role is to lower blood sugar to normal levels. It does this by moving sugar from the blood into cells, where it is used for energy. Think of insulin as a key that opens cell doors.

But if you have diabetes, either your body doesn't make enough insulin, or your cells don't respond to insulin.

This causes blood sugar to build up in your bloodstream, resulting in high blood sugar.

A diagnosis of diabetes means your pancreas can't make enough insulin to cope, and the result is an insulin deficiency. If your body can't produce enough insulin, your blood sugar levels become elevated. Long-term high blood sugar levels can affect almost every system in the body.

People with diabetes often think they need to focus strictly on avoiding sugar or carbohydrates and neglect to consider the nutritional quality of their diet. While it is true that carbohydrates have the greatest impact on blood sugar, it is the diet as a whole that contributes to health, weight management and blood sugar control. Strictly limiting the carbohydrates found in fruits and whole grains while eating a diet high in saturated fat and sodium does not promote optimal health.

Focusing on healthy foods, controlling carbohydrate portions, and losing weight if you are overweight are the three most important things you can do to manage type 2 diabetes from a nutritional standpoint. Limit your intake of added sugars, which are found in sugary drinks and many processed foods.

Breakfast Recipes

1. Creamed Spinach

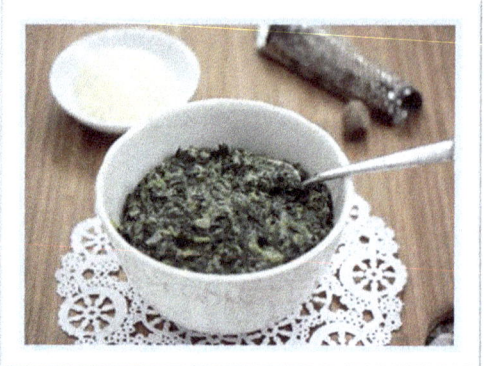

Preparation Time: 5 Minutes

Cooking Time: 10 Minutes

Effort: Easy

Servings: 4

Ingredients:

- 3 tbsp. Butter
- ¼ tsp. Black Pepper
- 4 cloves of Garlic, minced
- ¼ tsp. Sea Salt
- 10 oz. Baby Spinach, chopped
- 1 tsp. Italian Seasoning
- 1/2 cup Heavy Cream
- 3 oz. Cream Cheese

Directions:
1. Melt butter in a large sauté pan over medium heat.
2. Once the butter has melted, spoon in the garlic and sauté for 30 seconds or until aromatic.
3. Spoon in the spinach and cook for 3 to 4 minutes or until wilted.
4. Add all the remaining ingredients to it and continuously stir until the cream cheese melts and the mixture gets thickened.
5. Serve hot

Nutrition: Calories – 274kL; Fat – 27g; Carbohydrates – 4g; Protein – 4g; Sodium – 114mg

2. Stuffed Mushrooms

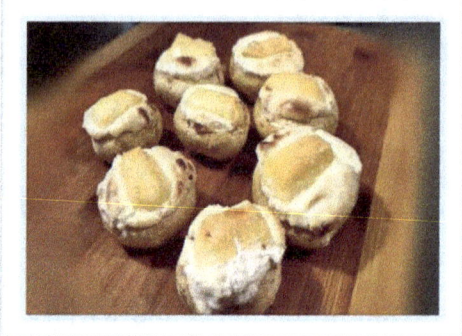

Preparation Time: 10 Minutes

Cooking Time: 20 Minutes

Servings: 4

Ingredients:

- 4 Portobello Mushrooms, large
- 1/2 cup Mozzarella Cheese, shredded
- 1/2 cup Marinara, low-sugar
- Olive Oil Spray

Directions:

1. Preheat the oven to 375 F.

2. Take out the dark gills from the mushrooms with the help of a spoon.

3. Keep the mushroom stem upside down and spoon it with two tablespoons of marinara sauce and mozzarella cheese.

4. Bake for 18 minutes or until the cheese is bubbly.

Nutrition: Calories – 113kL; Fat – 6g; Carbohydrates – 4g; Protein – 7g; Sodium – 14mg

3. Berry-Oat Breakfast Bars

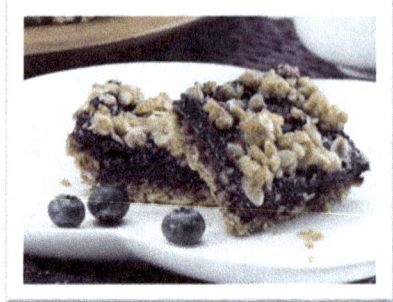

Preparation Time: 10 minutes

Cooking Time: 25 minutes

Servings: 12

Ingredients:
- 2 cups fresh raspberries or blueberries
- 2 tablespoons sugar
- 2 tablespoons freshly squeezed lemon juice
- 1 tablespoon cornstarch
- 11/2 cups rolled oats
- 1/2 cup whole-wheat flour
- 1/2 cup walnuts
- ¼ cup chia seeds
- ¼ cup extra-virgin olive oil
- ¼ cup honey
- 1 large egg

Directions:
1. Preheat the oven to 350f.
2. In a small saucepan over medium heat, stir together the berries, sugar, lemon juice, and cornstarch. Bring to a simmer. Reduce the heat and simmer for 2 to 3 minutes, until the mixture thickens.
3. In a food processor or high-speed blender, combine the oats, flour, walnuts, and chia seeds. Process until powdered. Add the olive oil, honey, and egg. Pulse a few more times, until well combined. Press half of the mixture into a 9-inch square baking dish.
4. Spread the berry filling over the oat mixture. Add the remaining oat mixture on top of the berries. Bake for 25 minutes, until browned.
5. Let cool completely, cut into 12 pieces, and serve. Store in a covered container for up to 5 days.

Nutrition: calories: 201; total fat: 10g; saturated fat: 1g; protein: 5g; carbs: 26g; sugar: 9g; fiber: 5g; cholesterol: 16mg; sodium: 8mg

30 minutes or less • nut free • vegetarian

4. Whole-Grain Breakfast Cookies

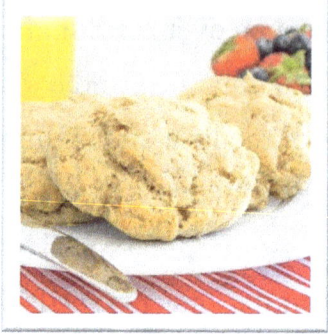

Preparation Time: 20 minutes
Cooking Time: 10 minutes
Servings: 18 cookies
Ingredients:
- 2 cups rolled oats
- 1/2 cup whole-wheat flour
- ¼ cup ground flaxseed
- 1 teaspoon baking powder
- 1 cup unsweetened applesauce
- 2 large eggs
- 2 tablespoons vegetable oil
- 2 teaspoons vanilla extract
- 1 teaspoon ground cinnamon
- 1/2 cup dried cherries
- ¼ cup unsweetened shredded coconut
- 2 ounces dark chocolate, chopped

Directions:
1. Preheat the oven to 350f.
2. In a large bowl, combine the oats, flour, flaxseed, and baking powder. Stir well to mix.
3. In a medium bowl, whisk the applesauce, eggs, vegetable oil, vanilla, and cinnamon. Pour the wet mixture into the dry mixture, and stir until just combined.
4. Fold in the cherries, coconut, and chocolate. Drop tablespoon-size balls of dough onto a baking sheet. Bake for 10 to 12 minutes, until browned and cooked through.
5. Let cool for about 3 minutes, remove from the baking sheet, and cool completely before serving. Store in an airtight container for up to 1 week.

Nutrition: calories: 136; total fat: 7g; saturated fat: 3g; protein: 4g; carbs: 14g; sugar: 4g; fiber: 3g; cholesterol: 21mg; sodium: 11mg

Appetizer Recipes

5. **Broccoli Salad**

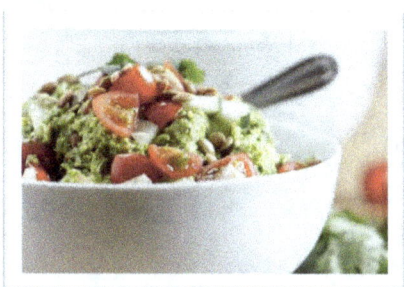

Preparation Time: 10 minutes

Cooking Time: none

Servings: 6

Ingredients:

- 1 medium head broccoli, raw, florets only
- 1/2 cup red onion, chopped
- 12 oz. turkey bacon, chopped, fried until crisp
- 1/2 cup cherry tomatoes, halved
- ¼ cup sunflower kernels
- ¾ cup raisins
- ¾ cup mayonnaise
- 2 tbsp. white vinegar

Directions:
1. In a salad bowl combine the broccoli, tomatoes and onion.
2. Mix mayo with vinegar and sprinkle over the broccoli.
3. Add the sunflower kernels, raisins and bacon and toss well.

Nutrition: Carbohydrates: 17.3 g; Protein: 11 g; Total sugars: 10 g; Calories: 220

6. Chicken Salad in Cucumber Cups

Preparation Time: 5 minutes

Cooking Time: 15 minutes

Servings: 4

Ingredients:

- 1/2 chicken breast, skinless, boiled and shredded
- 2 long cucumbers, cut into 8 thick rounds each, scooped out (won't use in a).
- 1 tsp. ginger, minced
- 1 tsp. lime zest, grated
- 4 tsp. olive oil
- 1 tsp. sesame oil
- 1 tsp. lime juice
- Salt and pepper to taste

Directions:

1. In a bowl combine lime zest, juice, olive and sesame oils, ginger, and season with salt.
2. Toss the chicken with the dressing and fill the cucumber cups with the salad.

Nutrition: Carbohydrates: 4 g; Protein: 12 g; Total sugars: 0.5 g; Calories: 116 g

7. Sunflower Seeds and Arugula Garden Salad

Preparation Time: 5 minutes

Cooking Time: 10 minutes

Servings: 6

Ingredients:

- ¼ tsp. black pepper
- ¼ tsp. salt
- 1 tsp. fresh thyme, chopped
- 2 tbsp. sunflower seeds, toasted
- 2 cups red grapes, halved
- 7 cups baby arugula, loosely packed
- 1 tbsp. coconut oil
- 2 tsp. honey
- 3 tbsp. red wine vinegar
- 1/2 tsp. stone-ground mustard

Directions:

1. In a small bowl, whisk together mustard, honey and vinegar. Slowly pour oil as you whisk.
2. In a large salad bowl, mix thyme, seeds, grapes and arugula.
3. Drizzle with dressing and serve.

Nutrition: Calories: 86.7g; Protein: 1.6g; Carbs: 13.1g; Fat: 3.1g

8. Supreme Caesar Salad

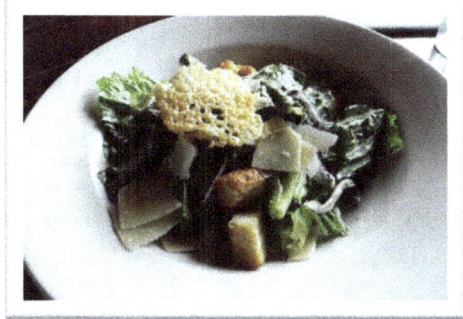

Preparation Time: 5 minutes
Cooking Time: 10 minutes
Servings: 4
Ingredients:
- ¼ cup olive oil
- ¾ cup mayonnaise
- 1 head romaine lettuce, torn into bite sized pieces
- 1 tbsp. lemon juice
- 1 tsp. Dijon mustard
- 1 tsp. Worcestershire sauce
- 3 cloves garlic, peeled and minced
- 3 cloves garlic, peeled and quartered
- 4 cups day old bread, cubed
- 5 anchovy filets, minced
- 6 tbsp. grated parmesan cheese, divided
- Ground black pepper to taste
- Salt to taste

Directions:
1. In a small bowl, whisk well lemon juice, mustard, Worcestershire sauce, 2 tbsp. parmesan cheese, anchovies, mayonnaise, and minced garlic. Season with pepper and salt to taste. Set aside in the ref.
2. On medium fire, place a large nonstick saucepan and heat oil.
3. Sauté quartered garlic until browned around a minute or two. Remove and discard.
4. Add bread cubes in same pan, sauté until lightly browned. Season with pepper and salt. Transfer to a plate.
5. In large bowl, place lettuce and pour in dressing. Toss well to coat. Top with remaining parmesan cheese.
6. Garnish with bread cubes, serve, and enjoy.

Nutrition: Calories: 443.3g; Fat: 32.1g; Protein: 11.6g; Carbs: 27g

9. Tabbouleh- Arabian Salad

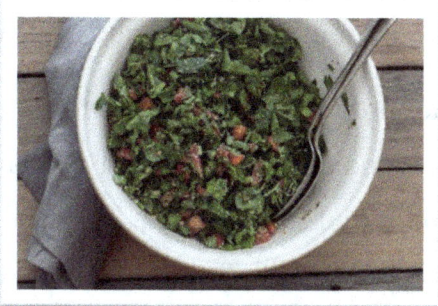

Preparation Time: 5 minutes

Cooking Time: 10 minutes

Servings: 6

Ingredients:
- ¼ cup chopped fresh mint
- 1 2/3 cups boiling water
- 1 cucumber, peeled, seeded and chopped
- 1 cup bulgur
- 1 cup chopped fresh parsley
- 1 cup chopped green onions
- 1 tsp. salt
- 1/3 cup lemon juice
- 1/3 cup olive oil
- 3 tomatoes, chopped
- Ground black pepper to taste

Directions:
1. In a large bowl, mix together boiling water and bulgur. Let soak and set aside for an hour while covered.
2. After one hour, toss in cucumber, tomatoes, mint, parsley, onions, lemon juice and oil. Then season with black pepper and salt to taste. Toss well and refrigerate for another hour while covered before serving.

Nutrition: Calories: 185.5g; Fat: 13.1g; Protein: 4.1g; Carbs: 12.8g

10.   Aromatic Toasted Pumpkin Seeds

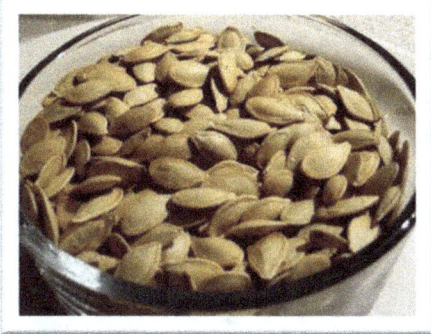

Preparation Time: 5 minutes
Cooking Time: 45 minutes
Serving: 4
Ingredients:

- 1 cup pumpkin seeds
- 1 teaspoon cinnamon
- 2 packets stevia
- 1 tablespoon canola oil
- ¼ teaspoon sea salt

Directions:

1. Prep the oven to 300°F (150°C).
2. Combine the pumpkin seeds with cinnamon, stevia, canola oil, and salt in a bowl. Stir to mix well.
3. Pour the seeds in the single layer on a baking sheet, then arrange the sheet in the preheated oven.

4. Bake for 45 minutes or until well toasted and fragrant. Shake the sheet twice to bake the seeds evenly.

5. Serve immediately.

Nutrition: 202 Calories; 5.1g Carbohydrates; 2.3g Fiber

11. Bacon-Wrapped Shrimps

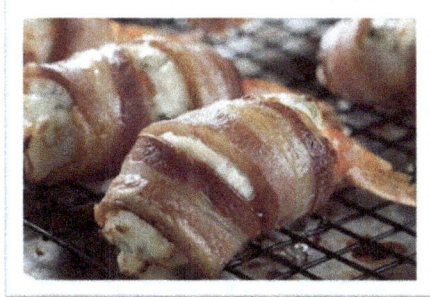

Preparation Time: 10 minutes

Cooking Time: 6 minutes

Serving: 10

Ingredients:

- 20 shrimps, peeled and deveined
- 7 slices bacon
- 4 leaves romaine lettuce

Directions:

1. Set the oven to 205°C.
2. Wrap each shrimp with each bacon strip, then arrange the wrapped shrimps in a single layer on a baking sheet, seam side down.
3. Broil for 6 minutes. Flip the shrimps halfway through the cooking time.
4. Take out from the oven and serve on lettuce leaves.

Nutrition: 70 Calories; 4.5g Fat; 7g Protein

First Course Recipes

12. Italian Beef

Preparation Time: 20 minutes

Cooking Time: 1 hour and 20 minutes

Servings: 4

Ingredients:

- Cooking spray
- 1 lb. beef round steak, trimmed and sliced
- 1 cup onion, chopped
- 2 cloves garlic, minced
- 1 cup green bell pepper, chopped
- 1/2 cup celery, chopped
- 2 cups mushrooms, sliced
- 14 1/2 oz. canned diced tomatoes
- 1/2 teaspoon dried basil
- ¼ teaspoon dried oregano
- 1/8 teaspoon crushed red pepper
- 2 tablespoons Parmesan cheese, grated

Directions:

1. Spray oil on the pan over medium heat.
2. Cook the meat until brown on both sides.
3. Transfer meat to a plate.

4. Add the onion, garlic, bell pepper, celery and mushroom to the pan.
5. Cook until tender.
6. Add the tomatoes, herbs, and pepper.
7. Put the meat back to the pan.
8. Simmer while covered for 1 hour and 15 minutes.
9. Stir occasionally.
10. Sprinkle Parmesan cheese on top of the dish before serving.

Nutrition: Calories 212; Total Fat 4 g; Saturated Fat 1 g; Cholesterol 51 mg; Sodium 296 mg; Total Sugars 6 g; Protein 30 g; Potassium 876 mg

13. Lamb with Broccoli & Carrots

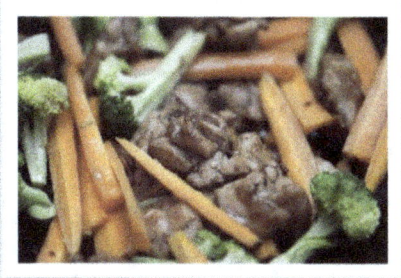

Preparation Time: 20 minutes
Cooking Time: 10 minutes
Servings: 4
Ingredients:

- 2 cloves garlic, minced
- 1 tablespoon fresh ginger, grated
- ¼ teaspoon red pepper, crushed
- 2 tablespoons low-sodium soy sauce
- 1 tablespoon white vinegar
- 1 tablespoon cornstarch
- 12 oz. lamb meat, trimmed and sliced
- 2 teaspoons cooking oil
- 1 lb. broccoli, sliced into florets
- 2 carrots, sliced into strips
- ¾ cup low-sodium beef broth
- 4 green onions, chopped
- 2 cups cooked spaghetti squash pasta

Directions:
1. Combine the garlic, ginger, red pepper, soy sauce, vinegar and cornstarch in a bowl.
2. Add lamb to the marinade.
3. Marinate for 10 minutes.
4. Discard marinade.
5. In a pan over medium heat, add the oil.
6. Add the lamb and cook for 3 minutes.
7. Transfer lamb to a plate.
8. Add the broccoli and carrots.
9. Cook for 1 minute.
10. Pour in the beef broth.
11. Cook for 5 minutes.
12. Put the meat back to the pan.
13. Sprinkle with green onion and serve on top of spaghetti squash.

Nutrition: Calories 205; Total Fat 6 g; Saturated Fat 1 g; Cholesterol 40 mg; Sodium 659 mg; Total Carbohydrate 17 g

14. Rosemary Lamb

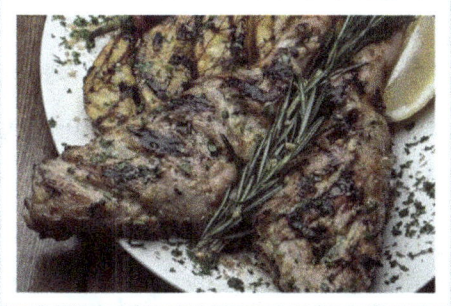

Preparation Time: 15 minutes

Cooking Time: 2 hours

Servings: 14

Ingredients:

- Salt and pepper to taste
- 2 teaspoons fresh rosemary, snipped
- 5 lb. whole leg of lamb, trimmed and cut with slits on all sides
- 3 cloves garlic, slivered
- 1 cup water

Directions:

1. Preheat your oven to 375 degrees F.
2. Mix salt, pepper and rosemary in a bowl.
3. Sprinkle mixture all over the lamb.
4. Insert slivers of garlic into the slits.
5. Put the lamb on a roasting pan.

6. Add water to the pan.

7. Roast for 2 hours.

Nutrition: Calories 136; Total Fat 4 g; Saturated Fat 1 g; Cholesterol 71 mg; Sodium 218 mg; Protein 23 g; Potassium 248 mg

15. Mediterranean Lamb Meatballs

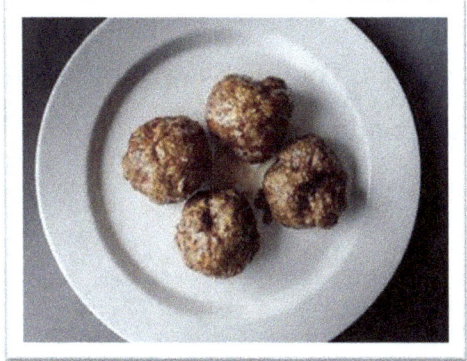

Preparation Time: 10 minutes

Cooking Time: 20 minutes

Servings: 8

Ingredients:

- 12 oz. roasted red peppers
- 1 1/2 cups whole wheat breadcrumbs
- 2 eggs, beaten
- 1/3 cup tomato sauce
- 1/2 cup fresh basil
- ¼ cup parsley, snipped
- Salt and pepper to taste
- 2 lb. lean ground lamb

Directions:

1. Preheat your oven to 350 degrees F.
2. In a bowl, mix all the ingredients and then form into meatballs.

3. Put the meatballs on a baking pan.

4. Bake in the oven for 20 minutes.

Nutrition: Calories 94; Total Fat 3 g; Saturated Fat 1 g; Cholesterol 35 mg; Sodium 170 mg; Total Carbohydrate 2 g; Dietary Fiber 1 g; Total Sugars 0 g

Second Course Recipes

16. Crab Frittata

Preparation Time: 10 minutes

Cooking Time: 50 minutes

Servings: 4

Ingredients:

- 4 eggs
- 2 cups lump crabmeat
- 1 cup half-n-half
- 1 cup green onions, diced

What you'll need from store cupboard:

- 1 cup reduced fat parmesan cheese, grated
- 1 tsp. salt
- 1 tsp. pepper
- 1 tsp. smoked paprika
- 1 tsp. Italian seasoning
- Nonstick cooking spray

Directions:

1. Heat oven to 350 degrees. Spray an 8-inch springform pan, or pie plate with cooking spray.

2. In a large bowl, whisk together the eggs and half-n-half. Add seasonings and parmesan cheese, stir to mix.

3. Stir in the onions and crab meat. Pour into prepared pan and bake 35-40 minutes, or eggs are set and top is lightly browned.

4. Let cool 10 minutes, then slice and serve warm or at room temperature.

Nutrition: Calories 276; Total Carbs 5g; Net Carbs 4g; Protein 25g; Fat 17g; Sugar 1g; Fiber 1g

17. Crunchy Lemon Shrimp

Preparation Time: 5 minutes
Cooking Time: 10 minutes
Servings: 4
Ingredients:
- 1 lb. raw shrimp, peeled and deveined
- 2 tbsp. Italian parsley, roughly chopped
- 2 tbsp. lemon juice, divided
- What you'll need from store cupboard:
- 2/3 cup panko bread crumbs
- 21/2 tbsp. olive oil, divided
- Salt and pepper, to taste

Directions:
1. Heat oven to 400 degrees.
2. Place the shrimp evenly in a baking dish and sprinkle with salt and pepper. Drizzle on 1 tablespoon lemon juice and 1 tablespoon of olive oil. Set aside.
3. In a medium bowl, combine parsley, remaining lemon juice, bread crumbs, remaining olive oil, and ¼ tsp. each of salt and pepper. Layer the panko mixture evenly on top of the shrimp.
4. Bake 8-10 minutes or until shrimp are cooked through and the panko is golden brown.

Nutrition: Calories 283; Total Carbs 15g; Net Carbs 14g; Protein 28g; Fat 12g; Sugar 1g; Fiber 1g

18. Grilled Tuna Steaks

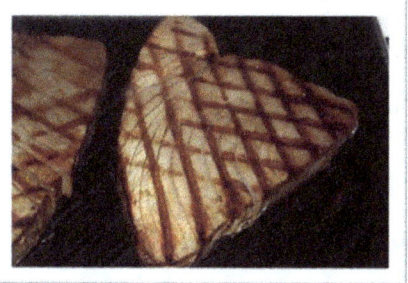

Preparation Time: 5 minutes

Cooking Time: 10 minutes

Servings: 6

Ingredients:

- 6 6 oz. tuna steaks
- 3 tbsp. fresh basil, diced
- What you'll need from store cupboard:
- 4 1/2 tsp. olive oil
- ¾ tsp. salt
- ¼ tsp. pepper
- Nonstick cooking spray

Directions:

1. Heat grill to medium heat. Spray rack with cooking spray.

2. Drizzle both sides of the tuna with oil. Sprinkle with basil, salt and pepper.

3. Place on grill and cook 5 minutes per side, tuna should be slightly pink in the center. Serve.

Nutrition: Calories 343; Total Carbs 0g; Protein 51g; Fat 14g; Sugar 0g; Fiber 0g

19. Red Clam Sauce & Pasta

Preparation Time: 10 minutes
Cooking Time: 3 hours
Servings: 4
Ingredients:

- 1 onion, diced
- ¼ cup fresh parsley, diced

What you'll need from store cupboard:

- 2 6 1/2 oz. cans clams, chopped, undrained
- 14 1/2 oz. tomatoes, diced, undrained
- 6 oz. tomato paste
- 2 cloves garlic, diced
- 1 bay leaf
- 1 tbsp. sunflower oil
- 1 tsp. Splenda
- 1 tsp. basil
- 1/2 tsp. thyme
- 1/2 Homemade Pasta, cook & drain

Directions:

1. Heat oil in a small skillet over med-high heat. Add onion and cook until tender, add garlic and cook 1 minute more. Transfer to crock pot.

2. Add remaining Ingredients, except pasta, cover and cook on low 3-4 hours.

3. Discard bay leaf and serve over cooked pasta.

Nutrition: Calories 223; Total Carbs 32g; Net Carbs 27g; Protein 12g; Fat 6g; Sugar 15g; Fiber 5g

20. Salmon Milano

Preparation Time: 10 minutes
Cooking Time: 20 minutes
Servings: 6
Ingredients:

- 2 1/2 lb. salmon filet
- 2 tomatoes, sliced
- 1/2 cup margarine

What you'll need from store cupboard:

- 1/2 cup basil pesto

Directions:

1. Heat the oven to 400 degrees. Line a 9x15-inch baking sheet with foil, making sure it covers the sides. Place another large piece of foil onto the baking sheet and place the salmon filet on top of it.

2. Place the pesto and margarine in blender or food processor and pulse until smooth. Spread evenly over salmon. Place tomato slices on top.

3. Wrap the foil around the salmon, tenting around the top to prevent foil from touching the salmon as much as possible. Bake 15-25 minutes, or salmon flakes easily with a fork. Serve.

Nutrition: Calories 444; Total Carbs 2g; Protein 55g; Fat 24g; Sugar 1g; Fiber 0g

21. Shrimp & Artichoke Skillet

Preparation Time: 5 minutes

Cooking Time: 10 minutes

Servings: 4

Ingredients:

- 1 1/2 cups shrimp, peel & devein
- 2 shallots, diced
- 1 tbsp. margarine

What you'll need from store cupboard:

- 2 12 oz. jars artichoke hearts, drain & rinse
- 2 cups white wine
- 2 cloves garlic, diced fine

Directions:

1. Melt margarine in a large skillet over med-high heat. Add shallot and garlic and cook until they start to brown, stirring frequently.

2. Add artichokes and cook 5 minutes. Reduce heat and add wine. Cook 3 minutes, stirring occasionally.

3. Add the shrimp and cook just until they turn pink. Serve.

Nutrition: Calories 487; Total Carbs 26g; Net Carbs 17g; Protein 64g; Fat 5g; Sugar 3g; Fiber 9g

22.   Tuna Carbonara

Preparation Time: 5 minutes

Cooking Time: 25 minutes

Servings: 4

Ingredients:

- 1/2 lb. tuna fillet, cut in pieces
- 2 eggs
- 4 tbsp. fresh parsley, diced

What you'll need from store cupboard:

- 1/2 Homemade Pasta, cook & drain,
- 1/2 cup reduced fat parmesan cheese
- 2 cloves garlic, peeled
- 2 tbsp. extra virgin olive oil
- Salt & pepper, to taste

Directions:

1. In a small bowl, beat the eggs, parmesan and a dash of pepper.

2. Heat the oil in a large skillet over med-high heat. Add garlic and cook until browned. Add the tuna and cook 2-3 minutes, or until tuna is almost cooked through. Discard the garlic.

3. Add the pasta and reduce heat. Stir in egg mixture and cook, stirring constantly, 2 minutes. If the sauce is too thick, thin with water, a little bit at a time, until it has a creamy texture.

4. Salt and pepper to taste and serve garnished with parsley.

Nutrition: Calories 409; Total Carbs 7g; Net Carbs 6g; Protein 25g; Fat 30g; Sugar 3g; Fiber 1g

23. Mediterranean Fish Fillets

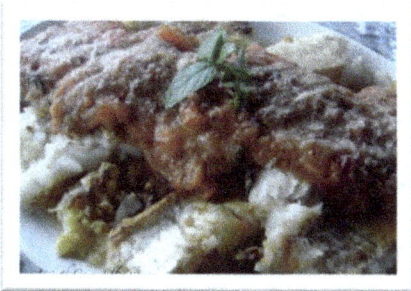

Preparation Time: 10 minutes

Cooking Time: 3 minutes

Servings: 4

Ingredients:

- 4 cod fillets
- 1 lb. grape tomatoes, halved
- 1 cup olives, pitted and sliced
- 2 tbsp. capers
- 1 tsp. dried thyme
- 2 tbsp. olive oil
- 1 tsp. garlic, minced
- Pepper
- Salt

Directions:

1. Pour 1 cup water into the instant pot then place steamer rack in the pot.
2. Spray heat-safe baking dish with cooking spray.

3. Add half grape tomatoes into the dish and season with pepper and salt.

4. Arrange fish fillets on top of cherry tomatoes. Drizzle with oil and season with garlic, thyme, capers, pepper, and salt.

5. Spread olives and remaining grape tomatoes on top of fish fillets.

6. Place dish on top of steamer rack in the pot.

7. Seal pot with a lid and select manual and cook on high for 3 minutes.

8. Once done, release pressure using quick release. Remove lid.

9. Serve and enjoy.

Nutrition: Calories 212; Fat 11.9 g; Carbohydrates 7.1 g; Sugar 3 g; Protein 21.4 g; Cholesterol 55 mg

Side Dish Recipes

24.   Chia Crackers

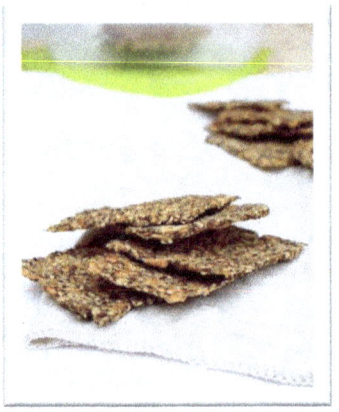

Preparation Time: 20 minutes

Cooking Time: 1 hour

Servings: 24-26 crackers

Ingredients:
- 1/2 cup pecans, chopped
- 1/2 cup chia seeds
- 1/2 teaspoon cayenne pepper
- 1 cup water
- 1/4 cup Nutritional yeast
- 1/2 cup pumpkin seeds
- 1/4 cup ground flax
- Salt and pepper, to taste

Directions:
1. Mix around 1/2 cup chia seeds and 1 cup water. Keep it aside.
2. Take another bowl and combine all the remaining Ingredients. Combine well and stir in the chia water mixture until you obtained dough.
3. Transfer the dough onto a baking sheet and rollout (¼" thick).
4. Transfer into a preheated oven at 325°F and bake for about half an hour.
5. Take out from the oven, flip over the dough, and cut it into desired cracker shape/squares.
6. Spread and back again for further half an hour, or until crispy and browned.
7. Once done, take out from oven and let them cool at room temperature. Enjoy!

Nutrition: 41 calories; 3.1g Fat; 2g Total Carbohydrates; 2g Protein

25. Orange- Spiced Pumpkin Hummus

Preparation Time: 2 minutes

Cooking Time: 5 minutes

Servings: 4 cups

Ingredients:

- 1 tablespoon maple syrup
- 1/2 teaspoon salt
- 1 can (16oz.) garbanzo beans,
- 1/8 teaspoon ginger or nutmeg
- 1 cup canned pumpkin Blend,
- 1/8 teaspoon cinnamon
- 1/4 cup tahini
- 1 tablespoon fresh orange juice
- Pinch of orange zest, for garnish
- 1 tablespoon apple cider vinegar

Directions:

1. Mix all the Ingredients to a food processor blender and blend until slightly chunky.
2. Serve right away and enjoy!

Nutrition: 291 Calories; 22.9g Fat; 15g Total Carbohydrates; 12g Protein

26.   Cinnamon Maple Sweet Potato Bites

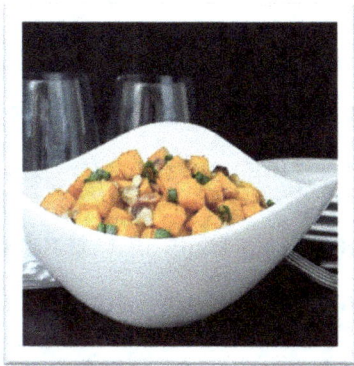

Preparation Time: 5 minutes

Cooking Time: 25 minutes

Servings: 3 to 4

Ingredients:

- ½ teaspoon corn-starch
- 1 teaspoon cinnamon
- 4 medium sweet potatoes, then peeled, and cut into bite-size cubes
- 2 to 3 tablespoons maple syrup
- 3 tablespoons butter, melted

Directions:

1. Transfer the potato cubes to a Ziploc bag and add in 3 tablespoons of melted butter. Seal and shake well until the potato cubes are coated with butter.
2. Add in the remaining Ingredients and shake again.

3. Transfer the potato cubes to a parchment-lined baking sheet. Cubes shouldn't be stacked on one another.

4. Sprinkle with cinnamon, if needed, and bake in a preheated oven at 425°F for about 25 to 30 minutes, stirring once during cooking.

5. Once done, take them out and stand at room temperature. Enjoy!

Nutrition: 436 Calories; 17.4g Fat; 71.8g Total Carbohydrates; 4.1g Protein

27. Cheesy Kale Chips

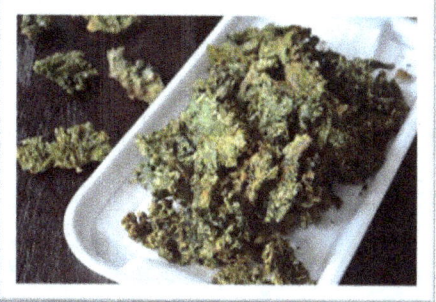

Preparation Time: 3 minutes

Cooking Time: 12 minutes

Servings: 4

Ingredients:

- 3 tablespoons Nutritional yeast
- 1 head curly kale, washed, ribs
- 3/4 teaspoon garlic powder
- 1 tablespoon olive oil
- 1 teaspoon onion powder
- Salt, to taste

Directions:

1. Line cookie sheets with parchment paper.
2. Drain the kale leaves and spread on a paper removed and leaves torn into chip-
3. towel. Then, kindly transfer the leaves to a bowl and sized pieces

4. add in 1 teaspoon onion powder, 3 tablespoons Nutritional yeast, 1 tablespoon olive oil, and 3/4

5. teaspoon garlic powder. Mix with your hands.

6. Spread the kale onto prepared cookie sheets. They shouldn't touch each other.

7. Bake into a preheated oven for about 350 F for about 10to 12 minutes.

8. Once crisp, take out from the oven, and sprinkle with a bit of salt. Serve and enjoy!

Nutrition: 71 Calories; 4g Fat; 5g Total Carbohydrates; 4g Protein

28.   Lemon Roasted Bell Pepper

Preparation Time: 10 minutes

Cooking Time: 5 minutes

Servings: 4

Ingredients:
- 4 bell peppers
- 1 teaspoon olive oil
- 1 tablespoon mango juice
- 1/4 teaspoon garlic, minced
- 1 teaspoons oregano
- 1 pinch salt
- 1 pinch pepper

Directions:
1. Start heating the Air Fryer to 390 degrees F
2. Place some bell pepper in the Air fryer
3. Drizzle it with the olive oil and air fry for 5 minutes
4. Take a serving plate and transfer it
5. Take a small bowl and add garlic, oregano, mango juice, salt, and pepper
6. Mix them well and drizzle the mixture over the peppers
7. Serve and enjoy!

Nutrition: Calories: 59 kcal; Carbohydrates: 6 g; Fat: 5 g; Protein: 4 g

29.   Subtle Roasted Mushrooms

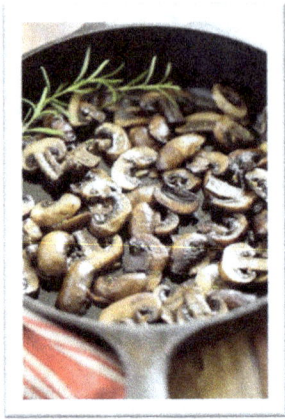

Preparation Time: 10 minutes

Cooking Time: 5 minutes

Servings:4

Ingredients:

- 2 teaspoons mixed Sebi Friendly herbs
- 1 tablespoon olive oil
- 1/2 teaspoon garlic powder
- 2 pounds mushrooms
- 2 tablespoons date sugar

Directions:

1. Wash mushrooms and turn dry in a plate of mixed greens spinner

2. Quarter them and put in a safe spot

3. Put garlic, oil, and spices in the dish of your oar type air fryer

4. Warmth for 2 minutes
5. Stir it.
6. Add some mushrooms and cook 25 minutes
7. Then include vermouth and cook for 5 minutes more
8. Serve and enjoy!

Nutrition: Calories: 94 kcal; Carbohydrates: 3 g; Fat: 8 g; Protein: 2 g

30. Fancy Spelt Bread

Preparation Time: 10 minutes
Cooking Time: 5 minutes
Servings:4
Ingredients:

- 1 cup spring water
- 1/2 cup of coconut milk
- 3 tablespoons avocado oil
- 1 teaspoon baking soda
- 1 tablespoon agave nectar
- 4 and 1/2 cups spelt flour
- 1 and 1/2 teaspoon salt

Directions:

1. Pre-heat your Air Fryer to 355 degrees F
2. Take a big bowl and add baking soda, salt, flour whisk well
3. Add 3/4 cup of water, plus coconut milk, oil and mix well
4. Sprinkle your working surface with flour, add dough to the flour
5. Roll well
6. Knead for about three minutes, adding small amounts of flour until dough is a nice ball

7. Place parchment paper in your cooking basket

8. Lightly grease your pan and put the dough inside

9. Transfer into Air Fryer and bake for 30-45 minutes until done

10. Remove then insert a stick to check for doneness

11. If done already serve and enjoy, if not, let it cook for a few minutes more

<u>Nutrition</u>: Calories: 203 kcal; Carbohydrates: 37 g; Fat: 4g; Protein: 7 g

31. Crispy Crunchy Hummus

Preparation Time: 10 minutes

Cooking Time: 10-15 minutes

Servings: 4

Ingredients:

- 1/2 a red onion
- 2 tablespoons fresh coriander
- 1/4 cup cherry tomatoes
- 1/2 a red bell pepper
- 1 tablespoon dulse flakes
- Juice of lime
- Salt to taste
- 3 tablespoons olive oil
- 2 tablespoons tahini
- 1 cup warm chickpeas

Directions:

1. Prepare your Air Fryer cooking basket
2. Add chickpeas to your cooking container and cook for 10-15 minutes, making a point to continue blending them every once in a while, until they are altogether warmed
3. Add warmed chickpeas to a bowl and include tahini, salt, lime

4. Utilize a fork to pound chickpeas and fixings in a glue until smooth

5. Include hacked onion, cherry tomatoes, ringer pepper, dulse drops, and olive oil

6. Blend well until consolidated

7. Serve hummus with a couple of cuts of spelt bread

Nutrition: Calories: 95 kcal; Carbohydrates: 5 g; Fat: 5 g; Protein: 5 g

Soups & Stews

32. Creamy Lentil and Potato Stew

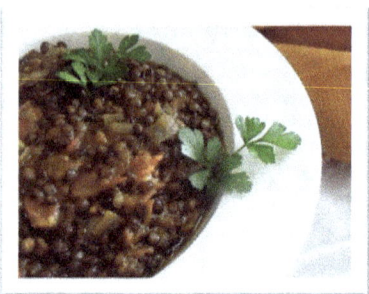

Preparation Time: 10 minutes

Cooking Time: 30 minutes

Servings: 4

This is a hearty stew that is sure to be a favorite. It's a one-pot meal that is the perfect comfort food. With fresh vegetables and herbs along with protein-rich lentils, it's both healthy and filling. Any lentil variety would work, even a mixed, sprouted lentil blend. Another bonus of this recipe: It's freezer-friendly.

Ingredients:

- 2 tablespoons avocado oil
- ½ cup diced onion
- 2 garlic cloves, crushed
- 1 to 1½ teaspoons sea salt
- 1 teaspoon freshly ground black pepper

- 1 cup dry lentils
- 2 carrots, sliced
- 1 cup peeled and cubed potato
- 1 celery stalk, diced
- 2 fresh oregano sprigs, chopped
- 2 fresh tarragon sprigs, chopped
- 5 cups vegetable broth, divided
- 1 (13.5-ounce) can full-fat coconut milk

Directions:

1. In a great soup pot over average-high hotness, heat the avocado oil. Include the garlic, onion, salt, and pepper, and sauté for 3 to 5 minutes, or until the onion is soft.

2. Add the lentils, carrots, potato, celery, oregano, tarragon, and 2½ cups of vegetable broth, and stir.

3. Get to a boil, decrease the heat to medium-low, and cook, stirring frequently and adding additional vegetable broth a half cup at a time to make sure there is enough liquid for the lentils and potatoes to cook, for 20 to 25 minutes, or until the potatoes and lentils are soft.

4. Take away from the heat, and stirring in the coconut milk. Pour into 4 soup bowls and enjoy.

Nutrition: Calories: 85; Carbohydrates: 20g; Fat: 3g; Protein: 3g

33. Roasted Garlic and Cauliflower Soup

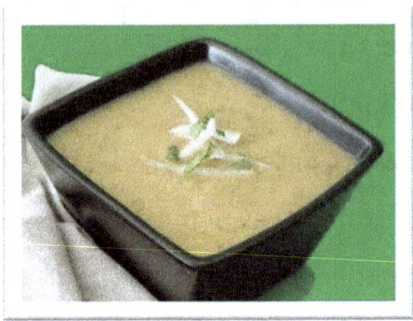

Preparation Time: 10 minutes
Cooking Time: 35 minutes
Servings: 1-2

Roasted garlic is always a treat, and paired with cauliflower in this wonderful soup, what you get is a deeply satisfy soup with savory, rustic flavors. Blended, the result is a smooth, thick, and creamy soup, but if you prefer a thinner consistency, just adds a little more vegetable broth to thin it out. Cauliflower is anti-inflammatory, high in antioxidants, and a good source of vitamin C (1 cup has 86 percent of your daily value).

Ingredients:
- 4 cups bite-size cauliflower florets
- 5 garlic cloves
- 1½ tablespoons avocado oil
- ¾ teaspoon sea salt
- ½ teaspoon freshly ground black pepper
- 1 cup almond milk

- 1 cup vegetable broth, plus more if desired

Directions:

1. Preheat the oven to 450°F. Line a baking sheet with parchment paper.

2. In a medium bowl, toss the cauliflower and garlic with the avocado oil to coat. Season with the salt and pepper, and toss again.

3. Transfer to the prepared baking sheet and roast for 30 minutes. Cool before adding to the blender.

4. In a high-speed blender, blend together the cooled vegetables, almond milk, and vegetable broth until creamy and smooth. Adjust the salt and pepper, if necessary, and add additional vegetable broth if you prefer a thinner consistency.

5. Transfer to a medium saucepan, and lightly warm on medium-low heat for 3 to 5 minutes.

6. Ladle into 1 large or 2 small bowls and enjoy.

Nutrition: Calories: 48; Carbohydrates: 11g; Protein: 1.5g

34. Beefless "Beef" Stew

Preparation Time: 10 minutes
Cooking Time: 0 minutes
Servings: 4

The potatoes, carrots, aromatics, and herbs in this soup meld so well together, you'll forget there's typically beef in this stew. Hearty and flavorful, this one-pot comfort food is perfect for a fall or winter dinner.

Ingredients:

- 1 tablespoon avocado oil
- 1 cup onion, diced
- 2 garlic cloves, crushed
- 1 teaspoon sea salt
- 1 teaspoon freshly ground black pepper
- 3 cups vegetable broth, plus more if desired
- 2 cups water, plus more if desired
- 3 cups sliced carrot
- 1 large potato, cubed
- 2 celery stalks, diced
- 1 teaspoon dried oregano
- 1 dried bay leaf

Directions:
1. In a medium soup pot over medium heat, heat the avocado oil. Include the onion, garlic, salt, and pepper, and sauté for 2 to 3 minutes, or until the onion is soft.

2. Add the vegetable broth, water, carrot, potato, celery, oregano, and bay leaf, and stir. Get to a boil, decrease the heat to medium-low, and cook for 30 to 45 minutes, or until the potatoes and carrots be soft.

3. Adjust the seasonings, if necessary, and add additional water or vegetable broth, if a soupier consistency is preferred, in half-cup increments.

4. Ladle into 4 soup bowls and enjoy.

Nutrition: Calories: 59; Carbohydrates: 12g

35. Creamy Mushroom Soup

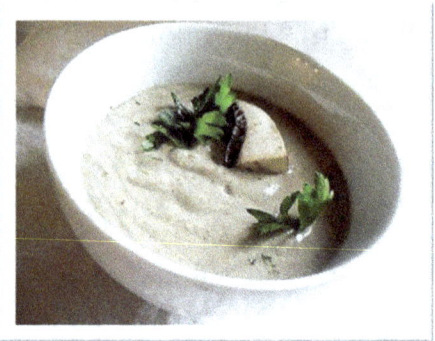

Preparation Time: 5 minutes

Cooking Time: 20 minutes

Servings: 4

This savory, earthy soup is a must try if you love mushrooms. Shiitake and baby Portobello (cremini) mushrooms are used here, but you can substitute them with your favorite mushroom varieties. Full-fat coconut milk gives it that close-your-eyes-and-savor-it creaminess that pushes the soup into the comfort food realm—perfect for those cold evenings when you need a warm soup to heat up your insides.

Ingredients:

- 1 tablespoon avocado oil
- 1 cup sliced shiitake mushrooms
- 1 cup sliced cremini mushrooms
- 1 cup diced onion
- 1 garlic clove, crushed
- ¾ teaspoon sea salt

- ½ teaspoon freshly ground black pepper
- 1 cup vegetable broth
- 1 (13.5-ounce) can full-fat coconut milk
- ½ teaspoon dried thyme
- 1 tablespoon coconut aminos

Directions:

1. In a great soup pot over average-high hotness, heat the avocado oil. Add the mushrooms, onion, garlic, salt, and pepper, and sauté for 2 to 3 minutes, or until the onion is soft.

2. Add the vegetable broth, coconut milk, thyme, and coconut aminos. Reduce the heat to medium-low, and simmer for about 15 minutes, stirring occasionally.

3. Adjust seasonings, if necessary, ladle into 2 large or 4 small bowls, and enjoy.

Nutrition: Calories: 65; Carbohydrates: 12g; Fat: 2g; Protein: 2g

36. Chilled Berry and Mint Soup

Preparation Time: 5 minutes

Cooking Time: 20 minutes

Servings: 1-2

There's no better way to cool down when it's hot outside than with this chilled, sweet mixed berry soup. It's light and showcases summer's berry bounty: raspberries, blackberries, and blueberries. The fresh mint brightens the soup and keeps the sweetness in check. This soup isn't just for lunch or dinner either—tries it for a quick breakfast, too! If you like a thinner consistency for this, just add a little extra water.

Ingredients:

FOR THE SWEETENER:

- ¼ cup unrefined whole cane sugar, such as Sucanat
- ¼ cup water, plus more if desired

FOR THE SOUP:

- 1 cup mixed berries (raspberries, blackberries, blueberries)
- ½ cup water
- 1 teaspoon freshly squeezed lemon juice
- 8 fresh mint leaves

Directions:
1. To prepare the sweetener

2. In a small saucepan over medium-low, heat the sugar and water, stirring continuously for 1 to 2 minutes, until the sugar is dissolved. Cool.

To prepare the soup:

3. In a blender, blend together the cooled sugar water with the berries, water, lemon juice, and mint leaves until well combined.

4. Transfer the mixture to the refrigerator and allow chilling completely, about 20 minutes.

5. Ladle into 1 large or 2 small bowls and enjoy.

Nutrition: Calories: 89; Carbohydrates: 12g; Fat: 6g; Protein: 2.2 g

37.   Vegetable Soup

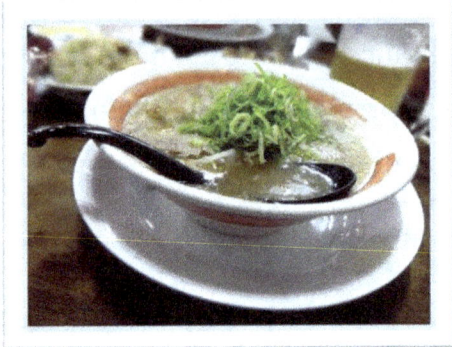

Preparation Time: 10 Minutes

Cooking Time: 30 Minutes

Servings: 5

Ingredients:
- 8 cups Vegetable Broth
- 2 tbsp. Olive Oil
- 1 tbsp. Italian Seasoning
- 1 Onion, large & diced
- 2 Bay Leaves, dried
- 2 Bell Pepper, large & diced
- Sea Salt & Black Pepper, as needed
- 4 cloves of Garlic, minced
- 28 oz. Tomatoes, diced
- 1 Cauliflower head, medium & torn into florets
- 2 cups Green Beans, trimmed & chopped

Directions:
1. Heat oil in a Dutch oven over medium heat.
2. Once the oil becomes hot, stir in the onions and pepper.
3. Cook for 10 minutes or until the onion is softened and browned.
4. Spoon in the garlic and sauté for a minute or until fragrant.
5. Add all the remaining ingredients to it. Mix until everything comes together.
6. Bring the mixture to a boil. Lower the heat and cook for further 20 minutes or until the vegetables have softened.
7. Serve hot.

Nutrition: Calories 79Kl; Fat 2g; Carbohydrates 8g; Protein 2g; Sodium 187mg

Desserts

38.   Walnut-Fruit Cake

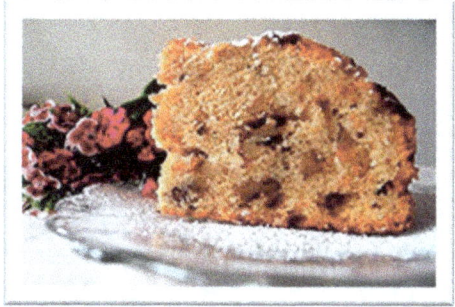

Preparation Time: 15 minutes

Cooking Time: 20 minutes

Servings: 6

Ingredients:

- 1/2 Cup of almond butter (softened)
- ¼ Cup of so Nourished granulated erythritol
- 1 Tablespoon of ground cinnamon
- 1/2 Teaspoon of ground nutmeg
- ¼ Teaspoon of ground cloves
- 4 Large pastured eggs
- 1 Teaspoon of vanilla extract
- 1/2 Teaspoon of almond extract
- 2 Cups of almond flour
- 1/2 Cup of chopped walnuts
- ¼ Cup of dried of unsweetened cranberries

- ¼ Cup of seedless raisins

Directions:

1. Preheat your oven to a temperature of about 350 F and grease an 8-inch baking tin of round shape with coconut oil.

2. Beat the granulated erythritol on a high speed until it becomes fluffy.

3. Add the cinnamon, the nutmeg, and the cloves; then blend your ingredients until they become smooth.

4. Crack in the eggs and beat very well by adding one at a time, plus the almond extract and the vanilla.

5. Whisk in the almond flour until it forms a smooth batter then fold in the nuts and the fruit.

6. Spread your mixture into your prepared baking pan and bake it for about 20 minutes.

7. Remove the cake from the oven and let cool for about 5 minutes.

8. Dust the cake with the powdered erythritol.

9. Serve and enjoy your cake!

Nutrition: Calories: 250; Fat: 11g; Carbohydrates: 12g; Fiber: 2g; Protein: 7g

39. Ginger Cake

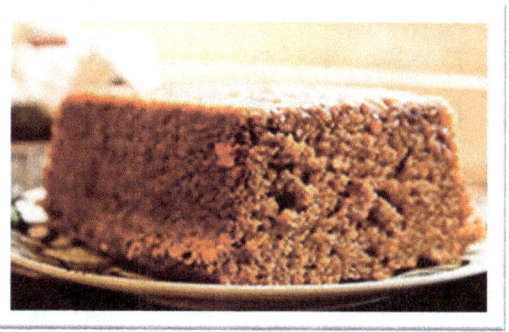

Preparation Time: 15 minutes
Cooking Time: 20 minutes
Servings: 9
Ingredients:

- 1/2 Tablespoon of unsalted almond butter to grease the pan
- 4 Large eggs
- ¼ Cup coconut milk
- 2 Tablespoons of unsalted almond butter
- 1 and 1/2 teaspoons of stevia
- 1 Tablespoon of ground cinnamon
- 1 Tablespoon of natural unweeded cocoa powder
- 1 Tablespoon of fresh ground ginger
- 1/2 Teaspoon of kosher salt
- 1 and 1/2 cups of blanched almond flour
- 1/2 Teaspoon of baking soda

Directions:

1. Preheat your oven to a temperature of 325 F.
2. Grease a glass baking tray of about 8X8 inches generously with almond butter.
3. In a large bowl, whisk all together the coconut milk, the eggs, the melted almond butter, the stevia, the cinnamon, the cocoa powder, the ginger and the kosher salt.
4. Whisk in the almond flour, then the baking soda and mix very well.
5. Pour the batter into the prepared pan and bake for about 20 to 25 minutes.
6. Let the cake cool for about 5 minutes; then slice; serve and enjoy your delicious cake.

Nutrition: Calories: 175; Fat: 15g ; Carbohydrates: 5g; Fiber: 1.9g; Protein: 5g

40. Ketogenic Orange Cake

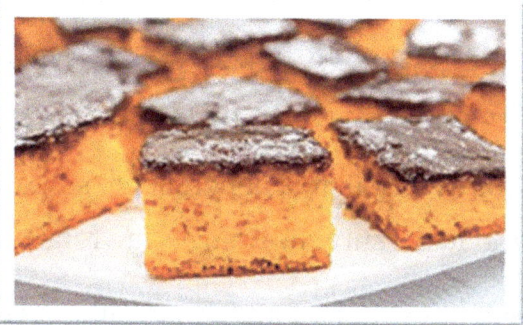

Preparation Time: 10 minutes

Cooking Time: 50minutes

Servings: 8

Ingredients:

- 2 and 1/2 cups of almond flour
- 2 Unwaxed washed oranges
- 5 Large separated eggs
- 1 Teaspoon of baking powder
- 2 Teaspoons of orange extract
- 1 Teaspoon of vanilla bean powder
- 6 Seeds of cardamom pods crushed
- 16 drops of liquid stevia; about 3 teaspoons
- 1 Handful of flaked almonds to decorate

Directions:

1. Preheat your oven to a temperature of about 350 Fahrenheit.

2. Line a rectangular bread baking tray with a parchment paper.

3. Place the oranges into a pan filled with cold water and cover it with a lid.

4. Bring the saucepan to a boil, then let simmer for about 1 hour and make sure the oranges are totally submerged.

5. Make sure the oranges are always submerged to remove any taste of bitterness.

6. Cut the oranges into halves; then remove any seeds; and drain the water and set the oranges aside to cool down.

7. Cut the oranges in half and remove any seeds, then puree it with a blender or a food processor.

8. Separate the eggs; then whisk the egg whites until you see stiff peaks forming.

9. Add all your ingredients except for the egg whites to the orange mixture and add in the egg whites; then mix.

10. Pour the batter into the cake tin and sprinkle with the flaked almonds right on top.

11. Bake your cake for about 50 minutes.

12. Remove the cake from the oven and set aside to cool for 5 minutes.

13. Slice your cake; then serve and enjoy its incredible taste!

Nutrition: Calories: 164; Fat: 12g; Carbohydrates: 7.1; Fiber: 2.7g; Protein: 10.9g

41. Lemon Cake

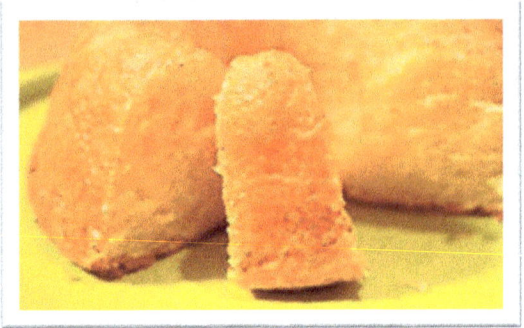

Preparation Time: 20 minutes

Cooking Time: 20minutes

Servings: 6

Ingredients:

- 2 Medium lemons
- 4 Large eggs
- 2 Tablespoons of almond butter
- 2 Tablespoons of avocado oil
- 1/3 cup of coconut flour
- 4-5 tablespoons of honey (or another sweetener of your choice)
- 1/2 tablespoon of baking soda

Directions:

1. Preheat your oven to a temperature of about 350 F.
2. Crack the eggs in a large bowl and set two egg whites aside.

3. Whisk the 2 whites of eggs with the egg yolks, the honey, the oil, the almond butter, the lemon zest and the juice and whisk very well together.

4. Combine the baking soda with the coconut flour and gradually add this dry mixture to the wet ingredients and keep whisking for a couple of minutes.

5. Beat the two eggs with a hand mixer and beat the egg into foam.

6. Add the white egg foam gradually to the mixture with a silicone spatula.

7. Transfer your obtained batter to tray covered with a baking paper.

8. Bake your cake for about 20 to 22 minutes.

9. Let the cake cool for 5 minutes; then slice your cake.

10. Serve and enjoy your delicious cake!

Nutrition: Calories: 164; Fat: 12g; Carbohydrates: 7.1; Fiber: 2.7g; Protein: 10.9g

42. Cinnamon Cake

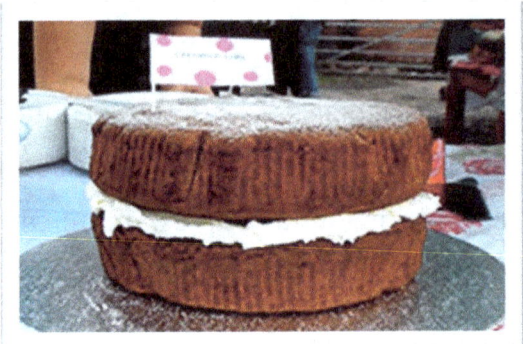

Preparation Time: 15 minutes

Cooking Time: 35 minutes

Servings: 6

Ingredients:

For the Cinnamon Filling:
- 3 Tablespoons of Swerve Sweetener
- 2 Teaspoons of ground cinnamon

For the Cake:
- 3 Cups of almond flour
- ¾ Cup of Swerve Sweetener
- ¼ Cup of unflavored whey protein powder
- 2 Teaspoon of baking powder
- 1/2 Teaspoon of salt
- 3 large pastured eggs
- 1/2 Cup of melted coconut oil
- 1/2 Teaspoon of vanilla extract

- 1/2 Cup of almond milk
- 1 Tablespoon of melted coconut oil

For the cream cheese Frosting:
- 3 Tablespoons of softened cream cheese
- 2 Tablespoons of powdered Swerve Sweetener
- 1 Tablespoon of coconut heavy whipping cream
- 1/2 Teaspoon of vanilla extract

Directions:

1. Preheat your oven to a temperature of about 325 F and grease a baking tray of 8x8 inch.

2. For the filling, mix the Swerve and the cinnamon in a mixing bowl and mix very well; then set it aside.

3. For the preparation of the cake; whisk all together the almond flour, the sweetener, the protein powder, the baking powder, and the salt in a mixing bowl.

4. Add in the eggs, the melted coconut oil and the vanilla extract and mix very well.

5. Add in the almond milk and keep stirring until your ingredients are very well combined.

6. Spread about half of the batter in the prepared pan; then sprinkle with about two thirds of the filling mixture.

7. Spread the remaining mixture of the batter over the filling and smooth it with a spatula.

8. Bake for about 35 minutes in the oven.

9. Brush with the melted coconut oil and sprinkle with the remaining cinnamon filling.

10. Prepare the frosting by beating the cream cheese, the powdered erythritol, the cream and the vanilla extract in a mixing bowl until it becomes smooth.

11. Drizzle frost over the cooled cake.

12. Slice the cake; then serve and enjoy your cake!

Nutrition: Calories: 222; Fat: 19.2g; Carbohydrates: 5.4g; Fiber: 1.5g; Protein: 7.3g

43.   Banana Nut Muffins

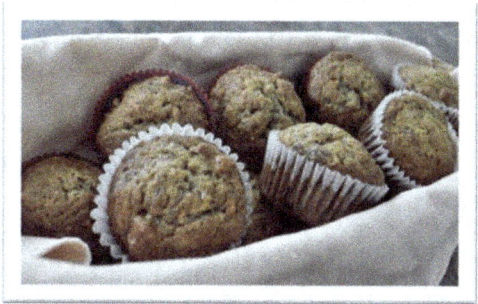

Preparation Time: 5 minutes

Cooking Time: 1 Hour

Servings: 6

Ingredients:

Dry Ingredients:

- 1 1/2 cups of Spell or Teff Flour
- 1/2 teaspoon of Pure Sea Salt
- 3/4 cup of Date Syrup

Wet Ingredients:

- 2 medium Blend Burro Bananas
- ¼ cup of Grape Seed Oil
- ¾ cup of Homemade Walnut Milk (see recipe)*
- 1 tablespoon of Key Lime Juice

Filling Ingredients:

- ½ cup of chopped Walnuts (plus extra for decorating)
- 1 chopped Burro Banana

Directions:
1. Preheat your oven to 400 degrees Fahrenheit.
2. Take a muffin tray and grease 12 cups or line with cupcake liners.
3. Put all dry Ingredients in a large bowl and mix them thoroughly.
4. Add all wet Ingredients to a separate, smaller bowl and mix well with Blend Bananas.
5. Mix Ingredients from the two bowls in one large container. Be careful not to over mix.
6. Add the filling Ingredients and fold in gently.
7. Pour muffin batter into the 12 prepared muffin cups and garnish with a couple Walnuts.
8. Bake it for 22 to 26 minutes until golden brown.
9. Allow to cool for 10 minutes.
10. Serve and enjoy your Banana Nut Muffins!

Nutrition: Calories: 150; Fat: 10 g; Carbohydrates: 30 g; Protein: 2.4 g; Fiber: 2 g

44.   Mango Nut Cheesecake

Cooking Time: 4 Hour 30 Minutes

Servings: 8 Servings

Ingredients:

Filling:

- 2 cups of Brazil Nuts
- 5 to 6 Dates
- 1 tablespoon of Sea Moss Gel (check information)
- 1/4 cup of Agave Syrup
- 1/4 teaspoon of Pure Sea Salt
- 2 tablespoons of Lime Juice
- 1 1/2 cups of Homemade Walnut Milk (see recipe)*

Crust:

- 1 1/2 cups of quartered Dates
- 1/4 cup of Agave Syrup
- 1 1/2 cups of Coconut Flakes
- 1/4 teaspoon of Pure Sea Salt

Toppings:

- Sliced Mango
- Sliced Strawberries

Directions:

1. Put all crust Ingredients, in a food processor and blend for 30 seconds.

2. With parchment paper, cover a baking form and spread out the blended crust Ingredients.

3. Put sliced Mango across the crust and freeze for 10 minutes.

4. Mix all filling Ingredients, using a blender until it becomes smooth

5. Pour the filling above the crust, cover with foil or parchment paper and let it stand for about 3 to 4 hours in the refrigerator.

6. Take out from the baking form and garnish with toppings.

7. Serve and enjoy your Mango Nut Cheesecake!

Juice and Smoothie Recipes

45. Strawberry – Orange Smoothies (SOS)

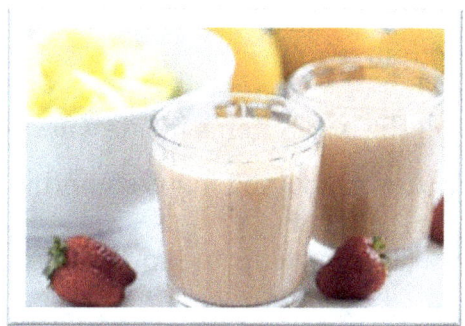

Preparation Time: 10 minutes

Cooking Time: 0 minutes

Servings: 1

Ingredients:

- 1 Cup Diced Strawberries
- 1 Removed Back of Seville Orange
- ¼ Cup Cubed Cucumber
- ¼ Cup Romaine Lettuce
- ½ Kelp
- ½ Burro Banana
- 1 Cup Soft Jelly Coconut Water
- ½ Cup Water
- Date Sugar.

Directions:
1. Use clean water to rinse all the vegetable items of ASOS into a clean bowl.
2. Chop Romaine Lettuce; dice Strawberry, Cucumber, and Banana; remove the back of Seville Orange and divide into four.
3. Transfer all the ASOS items inside a clean blender and blend to achieve a homogenous smoothie.
4. Pour into a clean big cup and fortify your body with a palatable detox.

Nutrition: Calories 298; Calories from Fat 9; Fat 1g; Cholesterol 2mg; Sodium 73mg; Potassium 998mg; Carbohydrates 68g; Fiber 7g; Sugar 50g

46. Tamarind – Pear Smoothie (TPS)

Preparation Time: 10 minutes
Cooking Time: 0 minutes
Servings: 1
Ingredients:

- ½ Burro Banana
- ½ Cup Watermelon
- 1 Raspberries
- 1 Prickly Pear
- 1 Grape with Seed
- 3 Tamarind
- ½ Medium Cucumber
- 1 Cup Coconut Water
- ½ Cup Distilled Water

Directions:

1. Use clean water to rinse all the ATPS items.

2. Remove the pod of Tamarind and collect the edible part around the seed into a container.

3. If you must use the seeds then you have to boil the seed for 15mins and add to the Tamarind edible part in the container.

4. Cubed all other vegetable fruits and transfer all the items into a high-speed blender and blend to achieve homogenous smoothie.

Nutrition: Calories: 199; Carbohydrates: 47 g; Fat: 1g; Protein: 6g

47. Currant Elderberry Smoothie (CES)

Preparation Time: 10 minutes
Cooking Time: 0 minutes
Servings: 1
Ingredients:
- ¼ Cup Cubed Elderberry
- 1 Sour Cherry
- 2 Currant
- 1 Cubed Burro Banana
- 1 Fig
- 1Cup 4 Bay Leaves Tea
- 1 Cup Energy Booster Tea
- Date Sugar to your satisfaction

Directions:
1. Use clean water to rinse all the ACES items
2. Initially boil ¾ Teaspoon of Energy Booster Tea with 2 cups of water on a heat source and allow boiling for 10 minutes.
3. Add 4 Bay leaves and boil together for another 4minutes.
4. Drain the Tea extract into a clean big cup and allow it to cool.
5. Transfer all the items into a high-speed blender and blend till you achieve a homogenous smoothie.

6. Pour the palatable medicinal smoothie into a clean cup and drink.

Nutrition: Calories: 63; Fat: 0.22g; Sodium: 1.1mg; Carbohydrates: 15.5g; Fiber: 4.8g; Sugars: 8.25g; Protein: 1.6g

48.   Sweet Dream Strawberry Smoothie

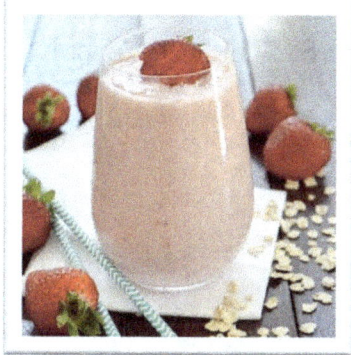

Preparation Time:1 5 minutes

Cooking Time: 0

Servings: 1

Ingredients:

- 5 Strawberries
- 3 Dates – Pits eliminated
- 2 Burro Bananas or small bananas
- Spring Water for 32 fluid ounces of smoothie

Directions:

1. Strip off skin of the bananas.
2. Wash the dates and strawberries.
3. Include bananas, dates, and strawberries to a blender container.
4. Include a couple of water and blend.

5. Keep on including adequate water to persuade up to be 32 oz. of smoothie.

Nutrition: Calories: 282; Fat: 11g; Carbohydrates: 4g; Protein: 7g

49. Alkaline Green Ginger and Banana Cleansing Smoothie

Preparation Time: 15 minutes

Cooking Time: 0

Servings: 1

Ingredients:

- One handful of kale
- one banana, frozen
- Two cups of hemp seed milk
- One inch of ginger, finely minced
- Half cup of chopped strawberries, frozen
- 1 tablespoon of agave or your preferred sweetener

Directions:

1. Mix all the Ingredients in a blender and mix on high speed.
2. Allow it to blend evenly.
3. Pour into a pitcher with a few decorative straws and voila you are one happy camper.
4. Enjoy!

Nutrition: Calories: 350; Fat: 4g; Carbohydrates: 52g; Protein: 16g

50. Orange Mixed Detox Smoothie

Preparation Time: 15 minutes

Cooking Time: 0

Servings: 1

Ingredients:

- One cup of vegies (Amaranth, Dandelion, Lettuce or Watercress)
- Half avocado
- One cup of tender-jelly coconut water
- One seville orange
- Juice of one key lime
- One tablespoon of bromide plus powder

Directions:

1. Peel and cut the Seville orange in chunks.
2. Mix all the Ingredients collectively in a high-speed blender until done.

Nutrition: Calories: 71; Fat: 1g; Carbohydrates: 12g; Protein: 2g

51. Cucumber Toxin Flush Smoothie

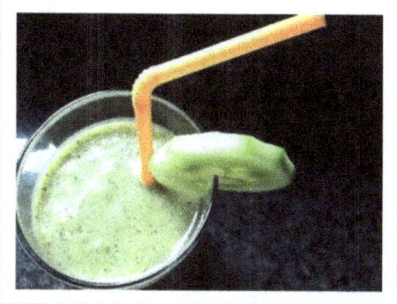

Preparation Time: 15 minutes

Cooking Time: 0

Servings: 1

Ingredients:

- 1 Cucumber
- 1 Key Lime
- 1 cup of watermelon (seeded), cubed

Directions:

1. Mix all the above Ingredients in a high-speed blender.
2. Considering that watermelon and cucumbers are largely water, you may not want to add any extra, however you can so if you want.
3. Juice the key lime and add into your smoothie.
4. Enjoy!

Nutrition: Calories: 219; Fat: 4g; Carbohydrates: 48g; Protein: 5g

Conclusion

Being diagnosed with diabetes will bring about some major changes in your lifestyle. From the moment you are diagnosed, it will always be a constant battle with food. You have to become much more mindful of your food choices and the amount you eat. Every meal will feel like a major effort to you. You will plan each day throughout the week well in advance. Depending on the type of food you ate, you need to keep checking your blood sugar levels. You may get used to taking long breaks between meals and not snacking between dinner and breakfast.

Managing diabetes can be a very, very stressful ordeal. There will be many times when you will mark your glucose levels on a piece of paper as if you are drawing graphic lines or something. You'll mix up your insulin shots and then you'll stress about whether you're giving yourself the right dosage. You will always be overly cautious because it's a lot of math and a very slim margin of error. But now, those days are over! If you start to notice that you are prediabetic or overweight, etc., there is always something you can do to change the situation.

Recent studies show that developing healthy eating habits and following low carbohydrate diets, losing excess weight and leading an active lifestyle can help protect you from developing diabetes, especially type 2 diabetes, by minimizing your risk factors for developing the disorder.

Too many carbohydrates can lead to insulin sensitivity and pancreatic fatigue, as well as weight gain with all the associated risk factors for cardiovascular disease and hypertension. The solution is to reduce your sugar intake, therefore, decreasing your body's need for insulin and increasing fat burning in your body.

When your body is low on sugars, it will be forced to use a subsequent molecule to burn for energy; in that case, this will be fat. The burning of fat will lead you to lose weight.

I hope you have learned something!

www.ingramcontent.com/pod-product-compliance
Lightning Source LLC
Chambersburg PA
CBHW070932080526
44589CB00013B/1485